MindBodyMed Press Mini-Monograph Series

THE EXPERIENCE OF BEING DIAGNOSED WITH CANCER

A PHENOMENOLOGICAL STUDY REVEALING THE LIVED-LIFE EXPERIENCES OF CANCER PATIENTS

KATHY BLOUGH, PSYS
Psychotherapist &
Certified Holistic Health Counselor

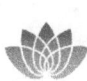

MindBodyMed
Press

Spring Lake | Michigan
United States

Publisher: MindBodyMed Press, LLC, PO Box 221
Spring Lake, Michigan, United States
www.MindBodyMedPress.com

Ordering Information:
Quantity sales. Special discounts are available on quantity purchases by corporations, associations, book clubs and others. For details, con-tact the publisher at the address above.

Publisher's Cataloging-in-Publication Data

Blough, Kathy.
    The Experience of being diagnosed with cancer : a phenomenologi-cal study revealing the lived-life experiences of cancer patients / Kathy Blough, Psy. S.
    p. cm.
    ISBN 9780615959665
    ISBN 9780990329701 (e-book)
    Includes bibliographical references.

1. Cancer --Diagnosis. 2. Cancer --Psychological aspects. 3. Holistic medicine. 4. Cancer --Patients. I. Title.
RC262 .B52 2014
616.99/4 --dc23   2014932136

MEDICAL DISCLAIMER

Health care is an ever-changing field. MindBodyMed Press, its editors, and authors of the mini-monographs, monographs, and creative nonfiction books have made every effort to provide information that is accurate and complete as of the date of publication and consistent with standards of good practice in the health care setting. As research and practice advance, however, standards may change. For this reason it is recommended that readers evaluate the applicability of any recommendations in light of particular situations and changing standards.

MindBodyMed Press mini-monographs, monographs, and creative nonfiction books are designed for educational purposes only and MindBodyMed Press, its editors and authors are not engaged in rendering medical advice or professional services. The information provided in this book should not be used for diagnosing or treating a health problem or a disease. It is not a substitute for professional care. Members of the public using this book are advised to consult with a physician regarding personal medical care. If you have or suspect you may have a health problem, consult your health care provider.

Although the author and publisher have made every effort to ensure that the information in this book was correct at press time, the author and publisher do not assume and hereby disclaim any liability to any party for any loss, damage, or disruption caused by errors or omissions, whether such errors or omissions result from negligence, accident, or any other cause.

Table of Contents

MindBodyMed
Press

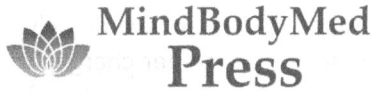

PUBLISHER'S WELCOME

While working on developing *MindBodyMed Press*, it became clear that *MindBodyMed Press* was going to become an indie publisher that would fill a void that exists in the way scientific information is shared with the public. The Internet has given everyone a voice as blogging platforms opened the door for anyone to spew words in digital format, making immediately available for public consumption any information, whether it is based on sound principles or mere ill-conceived opinions of self-appointed experts.

The National Center for Complementary and Alternative Medicine (NCCAM) draws attention to the problem in its Third Strategic Plan (2011-2015) in which the agency states that

> *Although a vast amount of information about CAM [Complementary and Alternative Medicine] is available in the public domain, much of it is incomplete, misleading, inaccurate, or based on scientifically unproven claims. Much of the public's use of CAM occurs in the absence of advice or guidance from health care providers (conventional or CAM)* (p. 14).

On the other extreme of the spectrum are peer-reviewed journals that serve the scientific community only.

Many of these traditional journals hide information behind well-gated databases, accessible only with costly annual subscriptions or per-paper charges that lie outside the pocketbooks of the average reader. One such example is a publisher who lists individual articles of a journal at a pay-per-view charge (access for 24 hours) at US $51 and unlimited access to said journal at an annual subscription of $1,038. The average per-article purchase price of another well-respected full-text scientific database is $35.95. *MindBodyMed Press's* titles are available for $7.99 and upwards in trade paperback and $6.99 and upwards in eBook format.

Falling in the middle are open-access peer review journals, which are free to consumers yet have a whole set of problems on their own, accepting bogus scientific research, seemingly more concerned with collecting hefty up-front charges from authors rather than helping the scientific community through peer review. For a thorough report on the state of affairs in the open-access scientific enterprise read "Who's Afraid of Peer Review?" by John Bohannon (2013). According to Bohannon, scientists agree that the open-access model itself is not to blame. One scientist describes the situation as not too much different than traditional subscription-based journals.

Despite this, the direction *MindBodyMed Press* is taking is no replacement for a thorough peer review in a reputable scientific journal. Scientific peer review, along with the cumbersome collection, interpretation, and reporting of data is necessary to inform health care providers, payers, employers, and patients of scientific data, allowing better evidence-based decision making pertaining to the use of mind-body interventions, practices, and disciplines.

However, peer review is usually a lengthy process and sometimes can take years.

Up until now, there has been no happy medium to afford the public access to the scientific literature. It simply is too expensive! Though things seem to be changing. The other day, while skimming The Chronicle of Higher Education, I came across an interesting article titled "The Rise of the Mini-Monograph" written by Leonardo Cassuto (2013).

A monograph, according to Merriam-Webster is "...a learned treatise on a small area of learning ... a written account of a single thing" (Merriam-Webster Dictionary, n.d.). Up until recently, a monograph was considered a one-volume work giving in depth treatment to a specialized subject, written by a scholar in the field, for mainly an academic audience (University of Illinois at Urbana-Champaign, n.d.).

According to Cassuto's (2013) article, however, several academic departments and scholarly presses are experimenting with shorter formats. Enter the mini-monograph. An entirely new book format, so to speak. The definitions from the previous paragraph still apply, though the length of the work is slightly smaller. Presses have begun using this new category to acquire and market original work. *MindBodyMed Press* is one of those presses.

Publisher Palgrave Pivot aims to attract original works between 30,000 and 50,000 words in length. Stanford Briefs publishes mini-monographs in the 20,000 to 40,000-word range. We at *MindBodyMed Press* believe that original works between 4,000 and 50,000 words, with

20,000-40,000 words being ideal, have considerable potential to reach a broad audience.

Like our counterpart Stanford Briefs, *MindBodyMed Press* believes that the purpose of making mini-monographs available to a wider audience is to foster "...an open argument rather than adding to a long conversation" (Cassuto, 2013). However, unlike Palgrave Pivot and Stanford Briefs, *MindBodyMed Press's* future lies in the integrative medicine niche market. According to NCCAM, practitioners integrating complementary and alternative medicine (CAM) for which there is some scientific evidence of safety and effectiveness into mainstream medicine are the key holders of knowledge related to the possible use of CAM in main stream medicine. These practitioners are in a good position to provide and share information that is of value to the public and health care providers (National Center for Complementary and Alternative Medicine, 2011).

What type of author should consider publishing with MindBodyMed Press and why?

MindBodyMed Press is a platform that allows practitioners embracing integrative medicine, be that medical doctors, nurses, nutritionists, CAM & mind- body medicine practitioners, and research scientists to connect with the public in a new format – the mini-monograph.

MindBodyMed Press closes the gap in the current publication process by changing the way integrative medicine practitioners communicate with the public, exposing their titles on mainstream platforms such as trade paperback and eBook (enhanced ePub v.3) publication through popular platforms such as Amazon.com, Kindle, Kobo, iBooks, etc. rather than specialized databases.

MindBodyMed Press aims for a quick turnaround: Less than three months from acceptance to publication in most cases.

Especially appealing to authors is that unlike traditional peer review publishing, the author retains copyright to their work. The author also receives royalties from the sale of their work. Yes! Unlike traditional peer review publishing, anytime an author's work is sold, he/she will receive royalties.

Publication with *MindBodyMed Press* is ideal for CAM and mind-body scientists, clinicians, and practitioners integrating those practices into mainstream medicine that do not want or do not need to subject themselves to a lengthy peer review process.

On the other hand, *MindBodyMed Press* also aims to be an indie publishing company for graduate students and junior faculty. According to Cassuto's article, Stephen Greenblatt, an American literary critic, theorist, and scholar at Harvard University, warned a decade ago not to force "…the most vulnerable members of the academic community - that is graduate students and junior faculty members - to fulfill outmoded requirements" (Cassuto, 2013). Cassuto continues to write that the best way to marshal in new practices is to support them.

At *MindBodyMed Press* we work closely with nonfiction authors, be that seasoned pros, or up and coming experts in the field of integrative medicine to create and share high quality information. In order for a manuscript to be considered for publication, authors must follow accepted scientific processes for original research (quantitative, qualitative, mixed methods research, reporting of case studies, and literature reviews) and/or best practices for nonfiction literary titles.

So, *MindBodyMed Press* will be adding quality CAM and mind-body medicine information from medical doctors, nurses, nutritionists, and research scientists to mainstream medicine. This information would have otherwise withered away on a researcher's or clinician's computer hard drive, never to see the light of day again, because it was either too long for peer review, and too short for a full length book.

Who do we serve?

MindBodyMed Press serves consumers who are curious about what the science says, as well as individuals with strong, often polar-opposite beliefs or biases regarding the state of evidence about CAM and mind-body interventions—or even the need for mind-body research.

MindBodyMed Press will present innovative new books, called mini-monographs, published to address the quintessence of a CAM or mind-body medicine modality. Mini-monographs are selected based on basic scientific criteria without sacrificing the quality of carefully edited and produced content. Mini-monographs will be published quickly promoting mindful, intelligent debate, while bringing novel perspectives and theoretical approaches within the reach of experts as well as the public.

MindBodyMed Press believes that you have a right to know what practitioners integrating CAM or mind-body modalities into mainstream medicine are doing right now to help people with their chronic ailments. If you are a cancer patient, you might not have years to wait for this process to play out in peer review. You need high quality information immediately in order to discern with your health care team if a CAM or mind-body modality might be beneficial in your particular case.

The only way this can happen is if you have access to timely information from the providers on the health care front, even if this information does not yet lead to conclusive evidence. Adhering to this publication model will allow *MindBodyMed Press* to put high quality integrative medical knowledge within economical reach of the public.

I am happy to share *MindBodyMed Press's* mission and vision with you here.

MindBodyMed Press's Vision:

> *Utilizing 21st century science and information technology, we will empower CAM practitioners, mind-body practitioners, clinicians, and scientists, who are the key holders of knowledge related to the potential use of mind-body interventions, to provide and share information that is of value to the public and to health care providers.*

MindBodyMed Press's Mission:

> *Given the reality of widespread and frequent self-care use of CAM and mind-body medicine,*

> *MindBodyMed Press will strive to share CAM and mind-body medical information primarily to health care consumers and health care providers who are curious about CAM and mind-body medicine, even when the evidence is inconclusive or does not lead to clear guidance.*

If you are a CAM or mind-body-oriented health care provider such as medical doctor, nurse, social worker, psychologist, research scientist, graduate student, nutritionist, etc., please consider submitting your finished manuscript to *MindBodyMed Press*. We especially want to hear from you if you have a manuscript pertaining integrating CAM, a mind-body modality, or a nutritional intervention pertaining to cancer. The only caveat; we will review your manuscript and make sure it adheres to accepted guidelines within the area of research in which your manuscript falls (quantitative research, qualitative research, mixed methods research, literature reviews, case studies, nonfiction, and so forth).

If you are a consumer in a bookstore skimming through this book, thank you for browsing, and I hope that the information contained meets your standards and you will consider purchasing this title. Purchasing a title not only provides you with solid information but a purchase also supports up-and-coming scholars (in many cases) in CAM, as well as practitioners and or researchers who have taken the time to share their experiences derived from many patient encounters or original research.

In return, we hope that if you are a consumer looking to address a health problem that the information contained herein will start a healthy dialogue between you, your primary health care provider(s), and your loved ones that takes into account your personal preferences.

Please do not hesitate to contact me should you have any further questions about your manuscript or the publishing process with *MindBodyMed Press*. If you are a health care consumer who has feedback on how to make *MindBodyMed Press* more appealing to you, I welcome your feedback as well.

Welcome to *MindBodyMed Press*. Your Mind. Your Body. Unite Them.

Werner Absenger
Managing Editor and Publisher MindBodyMed Press
werner@MindBodyMedPress.com

References:

Bohannon, J. (2013). Who's afraid of peer review?
    Science, 342(6154), 60–65.
    doi:10.1126/science.342.6154.60

Cassuto, L. (2013, August 12). The rise of the mini-
    monograph. *The Chronicle of Higher Education.*
    Retrieved from
    https://chronicle.com/article/The-Rise-of-the-Mini-
    Monograph/141007/

Identifying a scholarly monograph. (n.d.). Retrieved from
    University of Illinois at Urbana-Champaign website:
    http://www.library.illinois.edu/learn/research/
    monograph.html

Monograph. (n.d.). In *Merriam-Webster's online
    dictionary.* Retrieved from
    http://www.merriamwebster.com/dictionary/monograph

National Center for Complementary and Alternative
    Medicine. (2011). *NCCAM's Third Strategic Plan:
    Exploring the science of complementary and
    alternative medicine* (Third Strategic Plan).
    Retrieved from
    http://nccam.nih.gov/sites/nccam.nih.gov/files/
    NCCAM_SP_508.pdf

Author's Introduction

Being diagnosed with cancer is more than just a physical experience; it is a tumultuous psychological, emotional, and spiritual journey affecting every facet of one's life. The emotional impact of being diagnosed with cancer is often discounted or overlooked by medical professionals as well as by family members and friends of the patient. By not addressing the emotional component in the realm of cancer treatment, a significant part of the person goes unrecognized and untreated.

I have never been a cancer patient, but as a wife, daughter, granddaughter, niece, friend, and psychotherapist of those diagnosed, I have come to learn, personally and professionally, that treatment is far more than what is happening in the body. Successful treatment must encompass the whole person, including the mind and spirit; whether the outcome is life or death, the process by how the patient arrives at either destination is of utmost importance. It is my experience that friends and loved ones wish to help the patient, yet many do not understand the insidious role that cancer is playing in the patient's life. As a psychotherapist and student of mind-body medicine, it is my desire to enhance healing by highlighting the inseparable connection between the mind and body, and bring forth the emotional and psychological experiences of having cancer.

This study gives first-hand accounts of the experience of being diagnosed with cancer. I invite the reader to peruse the co-researcher's experiences and become aware of the themes that emerged from their interviews.

Lastly, I urge the reader to share the co-researcher's experiences with someone who has cancer, in an effort to open up a dialogue and explore with them "their experience of being diagnosed with cancer".

Sincerely,

Kathy Blough
Ann Arbor, Michigan
February 2014

MindBodyMed Press Mini-Monograph Series

THE EXPERIENCE OF BEING DIAGNOSED WITH CANCER

A PHENOMENOLOGICAL STUDY REVEALING THE LIVED-LIFE EXPERIENCES OF CANCER PATIENTS

KATHY BLOUGH, PSYS
Psychotherapist &
Certified Holistic Health Counselor

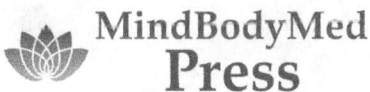

MindBodyMed
Press

Spring Lake | Michigan
United States

1

ABSTRACT

The purpose of this phenomenological pilot study was to investigate the experiences of people diagnosed with cancer. Three co-researchers, two men and one woman between the ages of 59-79, all diagnosed with cancer, were interviewed. Through these interviews, eight themes emerged depicting their emotional journey through cancer, which included, a) initial shock and denial, b) displaced anger, c) being self-absorbed, d) complying with and enduring treatment, e) fatigue, f) relationships, g) wanting to feel good again, and h) feeling alone – people didn't understand what they were enduring. While researchers in the scientific and medical communities are working to find ways to mend the body, understanding the emotional, intrapersonal, lived-life of the cancer patient is paramount for providing the necessary treatment and care to address healing on all levels of the cancer patient.

Keywords: cancer diagnosis,
cancer psychological aspects,
holistic medicine,
cancer patients,
phenomenology,
emotional experience

2

TOPIC INTRODUCTION

According to the National Cancer Institute (2012) nearly one in two men and women born in 2012 will be diagnosed with cancer some time during their lifetime. The National Cancer Institute estimates that "nearly 12 million Americans with a history of cancer were alive in January 2008" (p. 1). In 2012, approximately 1.6 million new cancer cases were expected to be diagnosed. Although cancer survival rates continue to increase each year, the rate of new occurrence is alarming. As cancer diagnoses continue to rise, the experience of being diagnosed with cancer will be an unfortunate yet common experience. While researchers in the scientific and medical communities are working to find ways to mend the body, understanding the emotional, intrapersonal, lived-life of the cancer patient is paramount for the whole person to heal and should be reflected in their medical treatment.

The purpose of this pilot study was to explore "what is the experience of being diagnosed with cancer?" The aim of studying this experience is to enhance healing by creating awareness and understanding, and by highlighting the impact that being diagnosed with cancer has on one's life and way of being-in-the-world. Understanding the breadth and depth of being diagnosed with cancer is critical to healing the whole being.

A cancer diagnosis can bring on a myriad of feelings including shock, trauma, denial, hopelessness, grief, fear, depression, and anxiety for the patient and their family (Kangas, Henry & Bryant, 2002; Kralik, Brown & Koch, 2001; Schæpe, 2011; Taylor, 2001). Rolland (1987) reports on the life cycle of a chronic illness from onset to outcome. He states that upon diagnosis, a system is created between the individual, their family, and their biopsychosocial systems. Rolland explores the interface between each of these systems and the reoccurring transitions that force change upon the individual, the family, and the biopsychosocial systems. The enormity of the impact to the individual's being and his or her way of life, especially in the initial stages of diagnosis, often creates a crisis in both the individual and the family. The crisis from family to family can vary, but can include an onset of intense emotions such as fear, loss, pain, encountering death, uncertainty, and financial concerns. These emotions, coupled with the integration of the hospital environment, disease-related treatment procedures, maintenance of family roles, and learning to deal with pain or incapacitation, can thrust a family into unchartered territory creating a crisis for the patient and family members.

Unfortunately, this crisis is often overlooked or denied by the medical profession as well as by extended family and friends. In 1994, with the introduction of the fourth edition of the Diagnostic and Statistical Manual for Mental Disorders (DSM-IV), being diagnosed with a life-threatening illness was finally recognized as a significant stressor that can precipitate post-traumatic stress disorder (Kangas,

Henry & Bryant, 2002). Given the prevalence and severity of cancer diagnoses, coupled with the likelihood of a crisis, it seems this experience would be well understood in the medical community and our culture at large. Yet, as a psychotherapist who has worked with individuals diagnosed with cancer, and as a daughter, granddaughter, niece, sister-in-law, friend, and wife of cancer patients, it is clear that the emotional devastation of this experience is still misunderstood and mostly ignored by the medical community and public at large. Therefore it is this researcher's desire to reveal the emotional and traumatic lived experiences of cancer patients in an effort to integrate these experiences into the matrix of treatment.

Depending on the onset of symptoms, the journey may begin prior to learning one has cancer, although diagnosis is the official starting point. At diagnosis, one's entire worldview will likely change; fear and uncertainty will form the foundation from which a new world-view will emerge. As Thorne, et al. (2010) reports, "regardless of the eventual outcome, hearing the news that one has cancer tends to become a new milestone within the life story, one that serves as a powerful reference point for making sense of past, present and future events" (p. 746). Candib (2004), a family physician who was diagnosed with a chronic illness, reports that words don't often represent the magnitude of the diagnosis experience. She writes:

> Coming to terms with 'being diagnosed,' 'having something,' needing to take daily medication or make permanent lifestyle changes, is a process that is not well understood by those who do the diagnosing. Although a MEDLINE term exists for this process-adaptation, psychological - the words do

" *not convey the turmoil and tortuosity of the experience (pp.148-149).*

For the cancer patient, the diagnosis is only the first step in a long journey riddled with turmoil, confusion, and pain. As Willig (2011) points out, at this phase of the epistemological journey the individual will have to "construct an entirely new identity for themselves (as 'cancer patient')" (p. 898). As one co-researcher expressed his new identity, he said, "I am now the weak one of the pack. I am not the rough and tough guy I always thought I was. I have become someone else, and I don't like it." From diagnosis onward, profound changes will occur in one's external and internal worlds and life will never return to pre-diagnosis days.

Being diagnosed with cancer, for most a life-threatening illness, is a complex, multilayered, life-changing event. It involves a reorganization of one's internal and external lives, a shattering of one's current world-view, and a creation and recreation of new world-views as the process unfolds. The illness trajectory is an on-going, arduous journey characterized by fear, loss, uncertainty, and pain. Being diagnosed is only the beginning of this life-altering event; enduring treatment and its aftermath also includes various bumps and pitfalls to be negotiated and endured.

3

Literature Review

Understanding the intrapersonal experience of the cancer patient can help to educate and guide the treatment of health care practitioners and enlist the help of family and friends of the cancer patient. Once diagnosed with cancer, communication with one's health care provider becomes of utmost importance and can impact the cancer patient's experience of the illness (Thorne, et al., 2010). To understand the impact that cancer care communication had between patients and their caregivers, Thorne, Hislop, Armstrong, and Oglov (2008) conducted individual interviews with a group of 200 patients. Sixty-nine individuals and 13 participants from a focus group all "explicitly identified communication as having an impact on their clinical outcomes, either positively or negatively" (p. 35). The authors note that although no clinical evidence of this phenomenon exists, many patients are convinced that communication with their health care professional is a critical factor in their treatment outcome and possibly linked to their survivorship. Aspects of positive communication with health care providers identified by patients included psychological comfort, perceiving themselves to be an active agent in their own care, and feeling hopeful.

In a small phenomenological study exploring the experience of being diagnosed with colorectal cancer, Taylor (2001) identified six themes and 15 sub-themes that emerged from the interviews of eight patients. The identified themes were: a) Making sense of the diagnosis, b) fearing the worst, c) redefining the future, d) having to go with the treatment, e) managing day-to-day, and f) feeling on their own (p. 655). These themes highlight the downward spiral that begins with diagnosis, including the loss of one's current world-view and the struggle to maintain life on all levels. As these themes revealed, the cancer patient's emotional needs go hand-in-hand with the process of medical treatment. These themes highlight the patient's lived-experience and reveal gaps in our medical system's realm of treatment. For the effective cancer treatment, Taylor suggests emotional support from family but also from volunteers who are patients themselves and have completed treatment. She suggests increased availability of nurses to provide the patient with information and guide them through the process from diagnosis to the completion of treatment.

Identifying coping strategies used at the time of diagnosis for women with breast cancer were found to be used throughout the cancer trajectory and attributed to enhanced meaning in life (Jim, Richardson, Golden-Kreutz & Andersen, 2006). Women who used active coping strategies along with social support at the time of diagnosis reported a greater sense of inner peace two years after diagnosis when compared with women who did not employ these strategies. When coping strategies of acceptance/positive reinterpretation and religious coping mechanisms were used at the time of diagnosis, these coping strategies also led to enhanced meaning in life, and higher scores in assessing life perspective, purpose, and goals.

In a phenomenological study entitled "Memories of Treatment: The Immediacy of Breast Cancer", author Thomas-MacLean (2004) explored the experience of breast cancer with 12 participants. All 12 women were between one and 24 years past their breast cancer diagnosis, however Thomas-MacLean found that memories of their treatment were articulated strongly and with much emotion. These emotional accounts indicated to the author that even though their treatments were completed, these past events were still being felt and experienced in the present. Five key themes that emerged through this study were: "(a) issues of control, (b) suffering, (c) encountering medicine, (d) visible loss, and (e) leaving active treatment" (p. 633). In conclusion, Thomas-MacLean reports that the concept of medicalization, defined as "the idea that some sort of tension exists between the acceptance of biomedical approaches, on one hand, and the critique of such approaches on the other" (p. 640), was woven throughout participants' treatment processes. The frustration of the objectification of their bodies and loss of autonomy throughout the process was coupled with the fear of severing ties with their biomedical practitioners. This dissonance was an underlying feature to the experience of suffering for many of the women in the study.

As shown by the above studies and supported by many others in the literature, communication, coping strategies, and the complicated emotional and psychological aspects of being diagnosed with cancer are at the forefront of the lived experience of cancer (Kangas, Henry & Bryant, 2002; Schæpe, 2011; Walsch & Nelson, 2003;

Willig, 2011; Winterbottom & Harcourt, 2004). Therefore, for treatment to be effective for the whole person, understanding associated behaviors and the psychological aspects that emerge from the cancer diagnoses are critical for treatment; however, most current models of treatment do not address the emotional or psychological aspects of this disease in their treatment protocols. Lee, Fitzgerald, Downey, and Moore (2012) report that although research has shown that treatment needs to be more comprehensive, innovative treatment has lagged behind. Overall, "the delivery of cancer care has not evolved to reflect the new realities of cancer survival and treatment complexity"... (p. 108).

In order to design effective cancer care models of treatment, it is critical to understand the lived experience of the cancer patient. This study is designed to reveal the emotional experiences of the cancer patient which, can in turn, highlight needed treatment areas. The next section provides an overview of the model used to explore the lived experiences of being diagnosed with cancer.

4

Overview of Research Model

Aphenomenological method of inquiry was used for further investigation into the experience of being diagnosed with cancer. Phenomenological research, as described by Creswell (2009), is "a strategy of inquiry in which the researcher identifies the essences of human experience about a phenomenon as described by participants" (p. 13). The phenomenological method of research is best used when it is important to develop a deeper understanding of an individual or several individual's experience of a phenomenon (Creswell, 2007). The phenomenological method of inquiry reveals the essential structure of the experience being investigated. This method of inquiry was chosen as a way to understand the experience of being diagnosed with cancer and to bring forth the meanings of such experience.

Once a question of social meaning and personal significance is formulated and a literature review is completed, the phenomenological process of data collection can begin (Moustakas, 1994). As a part of the data collection process, an internal inquiry is first conducted by the researcher using a process called epoche. Epoche is a Greek word meaning "refrain from judgment, to abstain

from or stay away from the everyday, ordinary way of perceiving things" (Moustakas 1994, p. 33). The purpose of
epoche is to clear the way for the researcher to gain new
insights into the human experience. Moustakas (1994) further explains:

> From the epoche, we are challenged to create new
> ideas, new feelings, new awarenesses and under-
> standings. We are challenged to come to know
> things with receptiveness and a presence that lets us
> be and lets situations and things be, so that we can
> come to know them just as they appear to us. (p. 86)

Although the concept is an ideal and cannot be really
fully reached (Creswell, 2007), engaging in the process can
help the researcher to release judgment, differentiate their
experiences from the co-researchers, and increase learning.

Once the researcher has engaged in epoche, the
process of collecting data from the co-researchers can
begin. In phenomenology, data is collected mainly
through interviews; however, observation, journals, poetry,
or art may also be used. The interview is usually informal,
interactive, and "utilizes open-ended comments and questions" (Moustakas, 1994, p. 14). The researcher creates a
climate in which the participant will respond comprehen-
sively and honestly. Questions are kept to a minimum, however they may be increased to facilitate a complete and rich
description of the phenomenon being studied. Interviews
are audio-recorded and transcribed for data analysis.

Data Analysis

Using a phenomenological hermeneutic approach to

data analysis, Lindseth and Norberg (2004) describe a method of interpretation designed to create movement between understanding and explanation. Their three-part process of data analysis consists of

1) conducting a naïve reading, whereas "the text is read several times to grasp its meaning as a whole" (p. 149). During this process, one attempts to switch their attitude from a natural state to a phenomenological attitude: that is, an attitude without judgment. The understanding that emerges from this first phase gives rise to the next stage of structural analysis.

2) Structural analysis is a method of interpretation whereas themes and sub-themes are identified through the extrapolation of meaning units and "reflected on against the background of the naïve understanding" (p. 150). During this phase the "what" of the experience emerges, giving way to the textual descriptions of the phenomenon, and the "how" the experience happened, or the structural descriptions, comes forth (Creswell, 2007).

3) Last is the comprehensive understanding or the interpreted whole. "The main themes, and sub-themes are summarized and reflected on in relation to the research question and the context of the study, i.e. the field of human life investigated" (Lindseth & Norberg, 2004, p. 150).

The results, or the lived-experiences, are presented in everyday language. The primary aim of this type of research is to

> *disclose truths about the essential meaning of being in the life world. We do not expect to find a*

> single fundamental truth; the whole truth can never be fully understood. We search for possible meanings in a continuous process. (Lindseth & Norberg, p. 151)

5

Methods

After formulating a question and conducting a literature review, participants (acknowledged throughout as co-researchers) were identified, data collection was obtained, and interviews were transcribed. The following paragraphs describe the participants and the analysis of the data.

Participants

Three co-researchers were interviewed in this pilot study. An open-ended, semi-structured interview format was used. Interview questions were kept to a minimum and are attached (see Appendix A). Interviews lasted between 70 and 90 minutes and were audiotaped and transcribed by this researcher. The co-researchers comprised two men and one woman ranging in age from 59 to 79; all are white and considered their economic status to be middle class. For confidentiality purposes, all names have been changed and identifying information has been omitted. The youngest, Mike, a 59-year-old man, has been known to this researcher for many years. He was diagnosed with Chronic Lymphocytic Leukemia (CLL) approximately two years ago and started chemotherapy two months prior to the interview. His cancer, CLL, is one of the cancers found to have been caused by exposure to Agent Orange. Mike is a Vietnam veteran and holds some resentment toward the military for his cancer diagnosis. He has been married for 30 years and has a 19-year-old son.

The second co-researcher, Brad, is an acquaintance and was referred by a friend of this researcher. He was diagnosed with Squamous Cell Carcinoma in November of 2011. Upon diagnosis, Brad had a tumor on the left side of his neck the size of a baseball. He is 65 years old, retired, twice divorced, and has one adult daughter and two grandsons. He currently lives alone. At the time of the interview Brad had completed three months of chemotherapy treatments and six weeks of daily radiation: His treatment protocol called for seven weeks of radiation but Brad decided he could not endure any more. He finished both treatments approximately four weeks prior to the interview.

Jan, the third participant, is a 79-year-old woman who was diagnosed with breast cancer in March of 2012. She was referred by a family member of this researcher and has known this researcher for many years. The participant and researcher had not had any contact for more than five years prior to the interview. She was diagnosed with breast cancer early in 2012 and had a double mastectomy in March of 2012. This was her second time being diagnosed with breast cancer; the first was 17 years earlier. Jan has been married for 55 years. She has three adult, male children, although one son died five years ago. In May of 2011 Jan lost her daughter-in-law to bone cancer and three days later her husband had heart surgery.

Interview Procedures

Upon being told about this study by various colleagues, friends, or family members, participants contacted this researcher indicating their interest in being a part of this study. An initial phone call was placed describing the study and a face-to-face interview was scheduled. Prior to the interview, this researcher engaged in the process of epoche on a number of occasions in order to release judgments and separate her personal experiences from the co-researchers.

The purpose of epoche as described by Moustakas (1994) is to clear the way for the researcher to gain new insights into the human experience. This process allows the researcher to be open to learning and to differentiate their experiences from the co-researchers. Although this researcher has never been diagnosed with cancer, she has been witness to friends, clients, and family members who have. To engage in epoche, this researcher focused on her private internal thoughts and feelings of the experience of being diagnosed with cancer. These experiences were recorded in a journal and numerous entries were made as private experiences emerged. Prior to each interview, this researcher engaged in a moment of meditation and deep breathing to clear away personal experiences and become open to the experiences of others.

During each meeting this researcher greeted her co-researchers and exchanged pleasantries; time was taken to create contact with each person. Before proceeding with the interview, this researcher explained the nature of the study and the interview process, and each participant was supplied with a packet of information which contained an explanation of the process in writing and the Consent to Participate form as provided by Saybrook University, San Francisco, California. The packet of information was reviewed with each participant. From there, a discussion ensued about the possibility of the emergence of painful feelings or memories during the interview process. This researcher conveyed permission for any and all emotions to surface and handed participants a card with the name and number of two area psychotherapists skilled at working with people diagnosed with cancer. Upon receipt of the cards and the information packet, questions were answered and the co-researchers signed the consent to participate.

The process started with sitting in silence for a few minutes. Each co-researcher was invited to take a few minutes to breathe evenly, and to settle into the present moment. Once each co-researcher indicated readiness to begin, the first of three questions was asked: "In thinking about your diagnosis of cancer, please describe your experience of being diagnosed with cancer and include your thoughts, what you said to yourself inside of your head, your feelings, and any sensations or reactions that you had as a result of your diagnosis."

Analyzing the Data

The data was analyzed using the hermeneutic phenomenological approached as described by Lindseth and Norberg (2004). First, this researcher performed a number of "naïve readings" of the transcripts, setting personal judgments aside in order to understand the meaning as a whole. The text was separated into meaning units and, through this process, themes and sub-themes emerged. Here the "how"- the structural descriptions- and the "what"- the textural descriptions of the experiences- came forth. These themes are presented and the verbatim passages from the co-researchers are given. Finally, a summary is presented, written in everyday language, to portray the co-researcher's experience of being diagnosed with cancer.

6

RESULTS

The themes that emerged as co-researchers detailed their experiences of being diagnosed with cancer were a) Initial shock and denial, b) displaced anger, c) being self-absorbed, d) complying with and enduring treatment, e) fatigue, f) relationships, g) wanting to feel good again, and h) feeling alone - people didn't understand.

Initial Shock and Denial

Upon being diagnosed with cancer, shock and denial were among the first responses that all three co-researchers mentioned. Each shared their experience when they were first diagnosed. Mike and Jan did not believe the diagnosis when first told, however each accepted it when further testing verified the initial findings. Brad doesn't remember when he was first diagnosed, however he didn't believe the diagnosis until he started his chemotherapy treatments. Mike's account of this experience was:

> *He [the doctor] said, "well the blood tests came back and indicated that you have"... he used a bunch of words, like carcinogen, lymphocytic, and all words like that, I knew them as individuals, but I*

> *didn't know them when you put them together, so I said, "what does all that mean?" He said, "it means you have cancer, you have chronic lymphocytic leukemia"… I remember when he said that, I had so much denial, I had a huge bulldozer of denial. I thought, "no, that's not true, I don't have cancer." It was kind of like a veil, a cloudiness was over me when he was talking… I remember I was thinking this next phrase to myself, I thought, "oh, the lab must have made a mistake". Then he responded to that statement… and I said, "did I say that out loud?" He chuckled and said, "yes, you did". I said, "I thought I was thinking it to myself." Then he responded, "they do make mistakes. They process millions of blood tests a year. So we are going to retest right now to make sure that it is accurate." But I just kept thinking, "no, I don't have cancer," then I went to the gym and worked out.*

Jan's experience of hearing she had cancer was similar.

> *When the doctor called me and told me I had cancer in the same breast as before, I was in shock, I couldn't believe it, I had very mixed emotions. I thought he doesn't know, they haven't done a biopsy yet so he might be wrong. I just kept thinking that. I also thought right away about my daughter-in-law who had died with bone cancer a year ago. At that time I thought, "why couldn't it be me? I had a good life, why her, she's so young?" Then when it happened to me I thought, "oh, I don't want this".… Also, you know when he [her doctor] called me and told me, he was in the airport. I heard all this noise and I asked him about it, he just said, "I'm*

> in the airport, on my way to"... wherever he was going, like it was just business as normal. I guess to him it was.

Brad's experience was somewhat different. He indicated that he vacillated between knowing and not knowing that he had cancer, but overall didn't believe it:

> I pretty much had an idea when I first went in because of the lump, but you know, you always hope, but... then after seeing my primary care doctor, he sent me to St. Joe's... and ya know, no one really said... Then when I went in to get my tonsils out because they were looking for the source of the lump, my sister was with me, and she asked the doctor directly, and he said yes, it was cancer, squamous cell or whatever it is called. So I just didn't know, it was so confusing, I just had a lot of doubt... no one had any good answers, I didn't believe I had cancer... actually maybe it was denial, I just don't know. [INTERVIEWER: "When do you think you really believed it?"] I don't really know, I still kind of don't believe it... maybe once I started doing chemo, or once the chemo started working and the lump started going away. People noticed it and said things to me about the lump looking better; I was shocked I didn't think anyone noticed it was even there, so when the chemo started working, I think maybe then... (laughter), I guess I had a lot of denial.

Displaced Anger

Displaced anger was a theme that occurred for all co-researchers shortly after diagnosis. Displacement as used in psychoanalytic theory and according to Oxford Diction-ary (2010) is "the unconscious transfer of an intense emo-tion from one object to another" (para. 3). All participants had an experience of displacing intense feelings, espe-cially anger, onto some other object. Jan shares her ac-count of displacement:

> To top it all off [after being diagnosed with breast cancer] I had this thing on my face, my doctor thought I should have it checked out, so I did. They called me and told me it was skin cancer and al-though I knew it wasn't nothing, it really bothered me. It was just skin cancer, I knew it wasn't life threatening, but it made me so mad, I just wanted to scream. I just wanted to go out into a field and scream. I can't tell you how mad I was about that spot on my forehead. Isn't that odd?

Brad experienced his feelings of displacement in a similar fashion. He reported:

> Ya know the thing that bothered me the most was learning that I was going to have to have all my teeth pulled out. I was so mad, it just hit me all at once. I was ok with everything until I went to the dentist. I was mad about that for a long time.

Mike's experience of displacement was towards the military. He stated:

> While I was in the doctor's office and he told me I had cancer, at the end of our conversation he rec-ommended I get an appointment with one of the

VA docs, since I was a Vietnam veteran. When I was leaving the doctor's, I just thought, "what the fuck, now I have to go back to the VA," the VA is military. It took me back to my history, back to the military. I was really pissed, and pissed at the military. You know, they actually include it [CLL] in a list of 10 diseases that is linked to Agent Orange, and they wouldn't admit to that if they didn't have overwhelming evidence. So, I felt pissed and again "used" like a stooge. I did a lot of stuff, training and stuff. When I came home I had to go to therapy to work out that stuff, but I thought I was done, just no more. I didn't want to go to the VA hospital, I wanted to go to my own private doctor or hospital, I didn't want to go to the VA, but I did. I wasn't really angry at the diagnosis, just at the military.

Being Self-Absorbed

The next theme that appeared was self-absorption. Each co-researcher described it in their own way, however collectively they experienced having difficulty thinking of anything but their cancer and themselves. Mike's report of this experience is as follows:

What's coming up for me now is this latest thing [chemo]. I had my first chemo treatment a month and a half ago and it brought it all forward again. I realize how much I am talking about it again... even when I am with friends, I realize I keep bringing the conversation back to me and what happened when I went through chemo that first time, and I have to do it again, five more times... it's all I think about and how I don't ever want to be inca-

> pacitated like that again. [Interviewer: "When you were first diagnosed, did you feel self-absorbed then too?"] Yes, I did. I just kept thinking about what was going on in my body, what I was going to do, and how mad at the military I was… you know, just knowing I have cancer, well, there is always this sense of heaviness with me, always, and I'm always thinking about it.

Brad reported he went vacillated among denial, not thinking about it at all, and being self-absorbed. His experiences were:

> At first I rarely thought about it. I had that lump on my neck in June. It was just small then, but I couldn't go to the doctor until I turned sixty-five and my Medicare kicked in. So I just didn't think about it. Then, after going to the doctors, it was all I could think about, plus you are constantly going to this doctor and that doctor… it's all you do, so it was all you can think about.

Jan reported feeling guilty about thinking about herself all the time. She said:

> It's all I could think about, I just thought about it all the time. I felt like "all I do is think about myself" and I didn't want to do that. I just thought about me all the time, I felt guilty about it, it was just always on my mind. I just dwelled on it. Especially in the beginning because I didn't know what was going to happen. I was wondering if I was going to have chemo. I knew I couldn't have radiation. I just didn't know what they were going to do, I was worried

> and scared and it was on my mind from the minute I woke up until I went to sleep.

Complying With and Enduring Treatment

The next phase that all co-researchers went through was treatment concerns. Mike and Brad did not want to have the recommended chemotherapy treatment while Jan felt grateful that she could have surgery and not radiation as she had 17 years ago.

Brad expressed it this way:

> I didn't want them to poison me with chemo and then fry me with radiation. They said they were going to give me three different kinds of chemo and then seven weeks of daily radiation... the radiation guy came in and started telling me all this stuff, like "we are going to radiate it [the tumor], the worst case scenario is we will have to give you a feeding tube cause you won't be able to eat cause your throat will be so sore, but it's no big deal. You know you will have to go to the dentist and have all your teeth out too, because after radiation on your neck and jaw you can't have any teeth problems because that would be very dangerous, you could lose your jaw bone." ... I just thought "What!? What is he talking about?" Feeding tube, teeth out? I was very scared, I didn't know what to do... After switching doctors and going to the UM [University of Michigan], I felt a little better, I know they ended up doing the same thing, they just presented it so much better, but I was still scared, really scared.... So before getting radiation and the

> chemo I had to have all my teeth pulled out, because the radiation can destroy your jaw bone and if your teeth are in bad shape like mine, you can actually lose your jaw bone, so they recommended I have all my teeth pulled. I couldn't get false teeth right away. So I still don't have any teeth. Then once treatment started the chemo wasn't so bad, it felt like I had a bad hangover for about four days, but it was the radiation that really got me. I was already losing some weight from the chemo, and not being able to eat much because I had my teeth out, but the radiation made it so I couldn't eat or drink hardly anything. I just felt terrible. I tried to gulp something down just to eat something, but I couldn't, my throat was like swollen, it felt plugged and it was sore, too. I just couldn't eat or even drink, and I was just going downhill every day. I had to go every day to have IV fluids. I got the radiation five days a week for six weeks. It really took all my energy. I didn't feel good and my neck was just awful, it was like raw meat; dead skin was everywhere, and it was really painful, I didn't know if I could tolerate much more.

Mike describes his experience of having to undergo chemotherapy two years after being diagnosed. At the point of our interview, he had one round of chemotherapy and would begin the second round in a couple of weeks. He was also scared about what might happen.

> I knew when I was getting worse and I might have to have chemo. I didn't want it though. I had read so many bad things about it and what happens to people having chemo. Six months ago I lost a dear

" *friend who had cancer and was undergoing chemo for about the third or fourth time. She had so many problems with it. I was really anxious about doing chemo, and probably the next time in a couple of weeks, I am probably going to be bursting at the seams, starting my second episode since the first episode just sucked. I felt feeble, weak, and I could not take care of myself. That's probably the first time that I couldn't take care of myself. I'm not at a point where I am dependent or that I can't take care of myself, however, while I was under the influence of chemo. I could not take care of myself. I could not even go to the store, I guess if I had too, I would have pushed, but I don't know if I would have passed out or not. Because just walking to the bathroom, my heart beat about ninety miles an hour…When I think about that first round of chemo, how sick I was, I remember I was just sitting on the floor with my bucket because if I moved at all my head would spin and I would either throw up or think I would throw up. I just kept telling myself "don't move." I then decided to just sit and stare at the fireplace, if I could just do that then time would pass, everyone said it's better in three to four days, so I thought I would just do that until then, but time felt like it wouldn't move. I just didn't know I was going to be incapacitated like that. I can get myself feeling really anxious just thinking about it. I think the treatment sucks, it's archaic, but it's the devil that I have to deal with right now.*

Jan's experience with undergoing treatment was a little different as she had surgery versus chemotherapy or radiation; nonetheless, her experience was scary for her as well:

> At the very beginning I was worried I might not make it. We were really worried because of my lungs, they didn't know if I would make it through the surgery because of my lungs. I have asthma and emphysema and the anemia. I had to have extra iron and stuff before the surgery. They were really worried about how long I could be under. When I asked about having both of them done [double mastectomy], Dave [her husband] was so worried I couldn't be under that long, but after they did all the tests and took precautions, they said it would be ok. We were both scared though.

Fatigue - Can't Engage in "Normal" Life

A theme that arose for all the co-researchers was how fatigued they felt, especially while going through treatment. They all shared how difficult the fatigue was and the frustration that they couldn't get back to living their normal life. Mike described it this way:

> One of my biggest challenges is being fatigued. I'm always tired. I can't exercise or do anything physical and I have always been physical. This coming weekend, I'm going to move my son out of his college dorm after completing his first year of school. Those are moments of excitement for me, but now it is like, I don't know if I can do it, I've always been pretty strong. Instead of going and grabbing a beer and making fun and yucking it up, I'm worried that I can't do much, and if I do, I've got to really monitor myself now, I can't be away from home long, it's limitations, I'm tired and I'm weak,

" *and I don't like it… I just want my life back… I want to feel normal and do my normal things.*

Jan described her experience of fatigue as:

" *I was just so tired, well I had anemia for three to four months before I was diagnosed, so I don't know if that is why I am still so tired, but I feel like I just can't do anything, and I'm even tired of that! [Laughter] Just so tired. Dave is so good he does everything, all the housework and everything and he's eighty-four years old! But I want to do stuff, but I can't. He gets worried when I want to do things, but I say I got to do stuff. I have to push some, and things got so out of hand over the last year, I haven't got done what I want done as far as clean-ing… Dave does very good, but…. It's not the same. I want to do it, but I just can't, and that bothers me.*

Brad's experience was:

" *When I was getting treatment, I just slept a lot, I couldn't do anything else, I was so tired. I couldn't go to the gym if I wanted to. I barely left the house, only for appointments and my sister came in to help me. I even needed her to drive me. Now that I think about it when I first started radiation, they would fit me with this big mask, and I would joke around with everyone, then, after a couple of weeks, I wouldn't say anything, I was too tired. Same with people in the waiting room, I met a lot of neat people in the waiting room. We were all going through and talking about the same thing. In the beginning I liked talking to these people but*

> by the end I didn't want to talk with anyone, it just really, really brought me down. [Interviewer: "In what way?"] Sickness, weak, I didn't want to talk with anyone, I just wanted to start feeling better again... I also lost weight, about fifty lbs, I couldn't eat or drink, it was just so hard then, everything was a chore, I just kept thinking, "I want to be normal again".

Relationships With Others

The role of relationships played a significant role for all three co-researchers. They all commented on the roles their loved-ones had in helping them endure their illness. All three commented on their trust or distrust of the medical professional involved in their care, and all mentioned how others just did not know what the experience of having cancer was really like for them. All three of them elaborated on their medical professionals' roles, therefore the relationships with medical professionals is listed as a sub-theme and elaborated on here.

- Medical Professionals

Jan reported feeling a great sense of trust in her physicians and medical practitioners. She stated she had positive feelings of caring and trust for them:

> My surgeon, Doctor, K., I didn't know her from before like I did the nurses, but she was so nice, whenever I see her, she gives me a hug, both when she sees me and when she leaves. [Interviewer: "What difference has that made for you?"] I think it's meant a lot to me, because she cared so much. When someone cares about you it means a whole

> lot, you are not just another number, and it's made me trust her. I really trust her and I feel safe with her. Even from the very beginning when they first said they were going to do surgery, she sat Dave and I down to talk with us about everything and one of the things she said was, "We had more to worry about than just the cancer." She was talking about doing the surgery with me having COPD, so I knew she was looking at everything and was concerned about it all.... I just had the nicest RNs, I still seem them sometimes. I saw one of them at Meijers last week and she gave me a big hug, she just cared. They were all really kind to me and I felt safe in their hands because of that.

Mike's experience was somewhat different, although he too trusted his physicians, which was important to him as well. He reported:

> I hated going to the VA hospital, but they have all treated me fine there. They have been kind and caring, except for one doctor I had. I don't think he ever even knew my name. I saw him for like three visits in a row; he was depressing, didn't offer hope, and talked about me as I was just a disease, like I [emphasis added] was cancer, not a person. Every time I left there after seeing him I felt worse, bad, kind of scared. Finally I decided I wouldn't see him anymore and I requested a new doctor. They gave me this small Jewish man. He was kind and caring, and talked to me, addressing me, and I liked him. I felt like he cared about me and what was happening to me. I'm glad I changed when I did, because that visit is when I learned they were

> recommending chemotherapy. At that point, I wasn't
> sure I was going to do it, but I had also just started
> working with another MD at an alternative medi-
> cine clinic. I really liked her. She had her foot in
> both worlds, alternative and traditional, and she
> was willing to help me. That felt good, like, "Ok, I
> got it now." I like using her for my guide. She said I
> needed to do the chemo, she said, "your numbers
> are so high, you got to do the chemo to bring you
> back to norm and from there we can take it, and I
> really believe you will be cancer free." So I did it. I
> did it because I trusted her. I also thought the new
> doc was trying to help me out, too, I just didn't
> know if I would go that route, but I am trusting they
> are going to help me.

Brad did not trust his physicians. His distrust added to his fear and frustration as he went through the treatment process. He shares:

> I just didn't know what to do. The radiation guy re-
> ally scared me. Doctor. H from St. Joe's said "Well,
> even if you go to the UM they will do the same
> thing, it's in the book, you look it up and it says
> chemo and seven weeks of radiation, that's how we
> treat it." I thought, what about me. I might be dif-
> ferent than others, I think we are all different and
> that we need individualized treatment. But I didn't
> trust him, he didn't have any good answers so I
> went to the UM and they wanted to do the same
> thing, right away. I said "No, we are just going to
> slow down, I am looking into alternative care." But
> they just wanted to do their stuff, poison me and
> fry me, I wasn't going to let them…. When my sister

> came to the doctor with me she asked them what
> would happen if I didn't treat it immediately. They
> said it would grow into my carotid artery and kill
> me…. I didn't want to believe that either, but she
> was pretty convinced after seeing the scans. So
> eventually I did it, after trying some alternative stuff
> that didn't really help, I decided I just had to get rid
> of that lump, so I did it, but it was scary, and I was
> angry about it… even when I went for chemo, my
> doctors weren't there, the nurses did everything. I
> don't think they knew what was going on.

Feeling Good Again

The desire to "feel good again" was a desire they all
experienced and mentioned numerous times throughout
their interviews. The chronicity of the illness and the treatment was difficult for all the co-researchers.

Brad shares:

> I was so sick of being sick that when I got up on
> that Monday of the seventh week of my radiation
> treatments, and I don't know where it came from,
> but I just decided, I'm done. I had one more week
> of radiation left, but I couldn't do it. My neck was
> raw, and I just couldn't go on like this anymore. I
> didn't think I would survive another week. I had to
> build my body back up, I just had to be able to feel
> good again and I knew I couldn't do that if I had
> any more radiation. I was afraid I would never feel
> good again if I didn't stop now, so I stopped it.

Jan reported:

> I just wanted to feel good again. When I had anemia then they found the cancer. I didn't know if I was going to ever feel good again. Even now it's hard, I was so tired with anemia which I had for five months prior to my surgery and now it's been over three months since I had my surgery and I'm still tired and really don't feel well yet. Ya know what helps though [Jan points to a picture located on her wall, it reads "Wine a little, you'll feel better"] [Interviewer: "A glass of wine?"] Yes, a glass or two of wine. Not every night or anything like that, but maybe if company stops over. It helps me to forget, to feel happy again, just for a moment in time.

Mike's desire to feel good again was described as:

> I was diagnosed over two years ago, and looking back on it I can see I had symptoms prior to that. I just didn't feel all that good. Over the two years I have been up and down, then six months ago, I just started going down and I haven't felt good since then. I really want to feel good again. They say the chemo will help my blood levels come back, and I know it's only been one out of six treatments, but so far, I'm not really feeling good yet. I just want to feel good again. I really want that back, to feel good and to have my life back.

Feeling Alone – People Didn't Understand

In closing the interview, the final question asked to each co-researcher was "What does it mean to you to be diagnosed with cancer?" Either in response to that question or when asked if there is anything else they wanted to share, all approached the subject of feeling alone with their cancer, stating that others didn't understand what they were really going through. Their responses are below.

Jan:

> Having cancer means you might die, and I had it twice and I didn't die, so I feel very fortunate in that respect, and fortunate for my doctors and my husband, and I feel that people just don't know. No one, unless it has happened to you, knows how traumatic it is to be diagnosed with cancer. People think you are just fine because you put a smile on your face and go into the grocery store, but you are not fine, they just don't get that, you could be dying. I had someone say to me, "Oh I knew you were feeling so much better because I saw you in the car with Dave out and about." What she didn't know was that I was just leaving the doctor's office from my check up and I was awful. I didn't like that she said I was just fine, I wasn't.

Brad:

> I didn't know what it meant, when all this started. I didn't know it was going to be like this. I didn't even know what an oncologist was. It all happened so fast, it was kind of surreal. It was like a dream, a bad dream…. I never thought I was going to die, I just didn't believe that, but I never thought it would be like this… and people just don't get it. They

"" don't have any idea what you are going through. They just don't know how bad it really is.

Mike:

"" It means I have a burden to carry that others don't. I've got to take care of it, heal it. I don't like it. It's like I got something that others' don't have, but I have got to deal with it. It separates me from the herd, so to speak. I am now the one that the lion is going to go after for meat. I am not the rough and tough guy that I thought I was... I may be again, but it separates me from the herd... I feel some of my friends are moving on and living and have kind of forgot me because I can't keep up with them, but, I'll be back. And there's a part of me that they don't know about, everything I go through. There's a part of me that wants to talk about it, like I want to talk about it on Facebook with some of my friends, but I don't think people want to hear it. I don't think they want to hear that I vomited for the fifth time after chemo. So they don't know, they think I am having a medical procedure, but I am going through trauma, again and again with this whole thing.

7

Summary & Conclusions

B eing diagnosed with cancer is a complex physiological and psychological experience, defined by pain, fear, uncertainty, trauma, shock, fatigue, anger, and denial. Varying levels of these emotions are felt throughout the cancer journey, a journey that can last for an undetermined amount of time. All three co-researchers shared how treatments from their area hospitals focused on their cancer and their biological needs, however none of their psychological needs were intentionally addressed. Any emotional needs that were met came indirectly from kindness and caring from their health care providers. Not feeling understood by family, friends, and medical personnel was a source of sadness and created a sense of loneliness for the participants.

The themes and emotional experiences of these three co-researchers indicate a desperate need for emotional support for cancer patients. The emotional turmoil and trauma experienced by cancer patients reveal the need to have access to on-going psychological support with trained and licensed psychological professionals throughout their cancer care. Patients need to be able to share their emotions, talk about their diagnoses, express their

anger, and learn coping and communication skills to effectively manage their emotions. This supportive, enhanced treatment approach can lead to reduced
emotional turmoil and can enhance the day-to-day lives
of people diagnosed with cancer.

8

LIMITATIONS OF RESEARCH

There were many limitations to this study, including group size, age group, and lack of diversity among co-researchers. In reviewing the transcripts, there are many areas where this researcher could have asked more questions to deeply explore many of the experiences the co-researchers were describing. A second interview would have also been helpful. Each participant was contacted by phone for follow-up questions and to inquire if they had anything further they would like to share. However, it is believed by this researcher that a second face-to-face conversation would have proven to be more valuable. Another limitation included the age of the participants. All co-researchers were 59 years of age or older and therefore did not have the added dimension of raising a family while going through this process. Two of the co-researchers were retired and also didn't have to think about job security. Only the youngest participant, Mike, brought up work and finances.

9

FURTHER RESEARCH

To extend this area of research and make use of these results, exploring models of care could be a valuable next step in addressing the psychological and emotional needs of the cancer patient. Through this study this researcher learned of the field "psycho-oncology". According to the International Psycho-Oncology Society (2010), which was founded in 1984, this organization was created to:

> Foster international multidisciplinary communication about clinical, educational and research issues that relate to the subspecialty of psycho-oncology and two primary psychosocial dimensions of cancer: 1) Response of patients, families and staff to cancer and its treatment at all stages; 2) Psychological, social and behavioral factors that influence tumor progression and survival. (para. 1)

A treatment model incorporating psycho-oncology practices into its treatment protocol could prove to be invaluable. All co-researchers were treated at leading hospitals for their cancer, however none of them were offered any counseling or psychological support during their treatment.

One patient, Brad, was treated at the University of Michigan hospital, which was ranked by U.S. News & World Report (2012) as the 14th best hospital in the nation for cancer care. Therefore, this researcher would wonder whether U.S. News & World Report does not understand or does not see treating psychological aspects of cancer as instrumental in its treatment. According to this small study, the psychological factors that coincide with having cancer are paramount in the day-to-day, lived experience of being diagnosed with cancer.

Finally, it is hoped by this researcher that this information, as well as other studies like it, can be imparted to health care providers to provide education and to create a network of care designed to support, educate, and heal on all levels, the patient diagnosed with cancer.

10

APPENDIX A

Interview Questions

According to the phenomenological method of research, questions are open-ended and kept to a minimum. The following questions served as a general structure for each of the individual interviews. Additional questions may be asked in order to encourage deeper exploration.

1. In thinking about your diagnosis of cancer, please describe your experience of being diagnosed and include your thoughts, (what you said to your self inside of your head), your feelings, and any sensations or reactions that you had as a result of your diagnosis.

2. What does it mean to you to be diagnosed with cancer?

3. Have you ever been diagnosed with cancer before?

Author's Suggested Reading & References

We ask the authors of our mini-monographs to provide a minimum of three titles of supplementary materials they consider essential reading pertaining the subject they wrote about. It is hoped that the mini-monograph you just read will have sparked your curiosity and interest for further study.

Ms. Blough suggests these titles:

Book List

Essential Reading:

Majors, C., Lerner, B., & Sayer, J. (2012) *The cancer killers: The cause is the cure.* Orlando, FL: Maximized Living.

Penzer, W. (2013). *How to cope better when someone you love has cancer.* Plantation, FL: Esperance Press, Inc.

Shapiro, D. (2013). *And in health: A guide for couples facing cancer together.* Boston, MA: Trumpeter Books

Supplemental Reading:

Mukherjee, S. (2010). *The emperor of all maladies: A biography of cancer.* New York, NY: Scribner

Bollinger, T. M. (2006). *Cancer: Step outside the box* (6th ed.). Infinity 510 Squared Partners

List of References

Candib, L. M. (2004). Making sense of my thumbs: Coming to terms with chronic illness. *Families, Systems, & Health,* 22(2), 139-151. doi:10.1037/1091-7527.22.2.139

Creswell, J.W. (2007). *Qualitative inquiry and research design: Choosing among five approaches.* (2nd ed.). Thousand Oaks, CA: Sage Publications.

Creswell, J. W. (2009). *Research design: Qualitative, quantitative, and mixed methods approaches* (3rd ed.). Thousand Oaks, CA: Sage Publications.

Home. (2010). Retrieved from International Psycho-Oncology Society website: http://www.ipos-society.org/

Jim, H. S., Richardson, S. A., Golden-Kreutz, D. M. & Andersen, B. L. (2006). Strategies used in coping with a cancer diagnosis predict meaning in life for survivors. *Health Psychology,* 25(6), 753-761. Retrieved from Academic Search Premier.

Kangas, M., Henry, J. L., & Bryant, R. A. (2002). Posttraumatic stress disorder following cancer: A conceptual and empirical review. *Clinical Psychology Review*, 22(4), 499-524.
doi:10.1016/S0272-7358(01)00118-0.

Kralik, D., Brown, M., & Koch, T. (2001). Women's experiences of "being diagnosed" with a long-term illness. *Journal of Advanced Nursing*, 33(5), 594-602. Retrieved from Acdemic Search Premier.

Lee, C. T., Fitzgerald, B., Downey, S., & Moore, M. (2012). Models of Care in Outpatient Cancer Centers. *Nursing Economics*, 30(2), 108-116. Retrieved from Academic Search Premier.

Lindseth, A., & Norberg, A. (2004). A phenomenological hermeneutical method for researching lived experience. *Scandinavian Journal of Caring Sciences*, 18(2), 145-153.
doi:10.1111/j.1471-6712.2004.00258.x

Moustakas, C. (1994). *Phenomenological research methods*. Thousand Oaks, CA: Sage Publications.

National Cancer Institute (2012). *Surveillance Epidemiology and End Results*. SEER Stat Fact Sheets: All Sites. Retrieved from
http://seer.cancer.gov/statfacts/html/all.html#risk

Displacement. (2010). *In Oxford Dictionaries*. (2010). Retrieved from
http://oxforddictionaries.com/definition/english/displacement

Rolland, J. S. (1987). Chronic Illness and the life cycle: A conceptual framework. *Family Process*, 26, 203-221. doi: 10.1111/j.1545-5300.1987.00203.x

Schæpe, K. S. (2011). Bad news and first impressions: Patient and family caregiver accounts of learning the cancer diagnosis. *Social Science & Medicine*, 73(6), 912-921. doi: 10.1016/j.socscimed.2011.06.038.

Taylor, C. C. (2001). Patients' experiences of "feeling on their own" following a diagnosis of colorectal cancer: A phenomenological approach. *International Journal of Nursing Studies*, 38(6), 651-661. doi:10.1016/S0020-7489(00)00109-7

Thomas-MacLean, R. (2004). Memories of treatment: The immediacy of breast cancer. *Qualitative Health Research*, 14(5), 628-643. doi:10.1177/1049732304263658

Thorne S., Oliffe, J., Kim-Sing, C., Hislop, T. G., Stajduhar, K., Harris, S. R., … Oglov, V. (2010). Helpful communications during the diagnostic period: An interpretive description of patient preferences. *European Journal of Cancer Care*, 19(6), 746-754. doi:10.1111/j.1365-2354.2009.01125.x

Thorne, S. E., Hislop, T., Armstrong, E., & Oglov, V. (2008). Cancer care communication: The power to harm and the power to heal? *Patient Education and Counseling*, 71(1), 34-40. doi:10.1016/j.pec.2007.11.010

Best hospitals: Cancer. (2012). Retrieved from U. S. News & World Report website: http://health.usnews.com/besthospitals/rank ings/cancer?page=2

Walsh, D., & Nelson, K. A. (2003). Communication of a cancer diagnosis: Patients' perceptions of when they were first told they had cancer. *American Journal of Hospice & Palliative Care*, 20(1), 52-56. doi:10.1177/104990910302000112

Willig, C. (2011). Cancer diagnosis as discursive capture: Phenomenological repercussions of being posi- tioned within dominant constructions of cancer. *Social Science & Medicine*, 73,(6). 897-903, doi:10.1016/j.socscimed.2011.02.028

Winterbottom, A., & Harcourt, D. (2004). Patients' experience of the diagnosis and treatment of skin cancer. *Journal of Advanced Nursing*, 48(3), 226- 233. doi:10.1111/j.1365-2648.2004.03191.x

AFTERWORD

MindBodyMed Press's Manuscript Review

Introduction

The Eight-Fold Path to a Publishable Mini-Monograph

All manuscripts received are reviewed by the managing editor based on MindBodyMed Press's "Eight-Fold Path to a Publishable Mini-Monograph."

This evaluation process allows us to appraise all manuscripts we receive based on the same basic quality guidelines. Once a manuscript passes all eight checkpoints, we believe that we have a high-quality mini-monograph on our hands. Such a mini-monograph has the potential to add additional quality information to the field of CAM and mind-body medicine, filling a void that currently exists in the way sharing of scientific information occurs with the public.

A brief overview of our evaluation criteria, along with an explanation of each item, follows.

1. Quality of design and methods
2. Clarity and readability
3. Literature review and use of references
4. Adequate data analyses
5. Rationale and theoretical development of hypotheses
6. Legitimacy of conclusions
7. Quality of discussion
8. Contributes new knowledge in the field

1. Quality of Design and Methods

Good guidelines exist for almost any type of research. The design and methods will vary with type of study. We want to know if reporting in the mini-monograph is based on generally accepted methods of scientific research in the field the author engages in. This will give a picture of reliability and validity of the reporting in the mini-monograph (American Psychological Association, 2010).

2. Clarity and Readability

Here, we look for whether the manuscript is the optimal length to allow the author to communicate effectively the primary ideas elaborated on in the mini-monograph. Does the structure of the mini-monograph help develop the argument? Are headings and paragraphs, lists, tables, numbering used appropriately? Are ideas presented so they can be followed easily? How about smoothness of expression? Does the text flow easily and effortlessly? Is the author's tone appropriate for the manuscript? Is the author communicating with precision and clarity? Does the author avoid bias? Does the author communicate with an educated lay audience in mind (American Psychological Association, 2010)?

3. Literature Review and Use of References

A literature review discusses written knowledge in a distinct subject area. A literature review may be only a mere summary of the references, but it customarily has an organizational pattern and consolidates both summary and synthesis. A summary is a recap of the essential knowledge of the source, but a synthesis is a re-organization of that information. It might provide a brand-new appreciation of old material or blend new with old themes. A literature review might ascertain the intellectual progress of the field, covering major debates (University of North Carolina, n.d.).

The literature review may assess the sources and inform the reader on the most appropriate or applicable sources pertaining a subject area. In a research paper, one applies the literature as a basis and support for a novel idea that the author has (University of North Carolina, n.d.).

For research falling into the realm of quantitative literature reviews and research papers employing a quantitative methodology, we evaluate literature reviews based on The PRISMA Statement: The Preferred Reporting System for Systematic Reviews and Meta-Analyses (Liberati et al., 2009).

For a study, that involves mainly qualitative research, we evaluate the literature reviews based on Noblit and Hare (1998), Ogawa and Malen (1992) and Gall, Borg and Gall (1996). Evaluating literature reviews for phenomenological studies we look for guidance to Moustakas (1994).

Boote and Beile's (2005) Literature Review Scoring Rubric highlights key points we seek out in a literature review, regardless of the investigation's methodology.

We also want to know whether the author cites relevant material. Do those citations provide enough background information to support the author's hypothesis? Do the citations place the author's contribution to the field in the context? Is each key point supported with a minimum of one or two sources that are most representative of that key point (American Psychological Association, 2010)?

4. Adequate Data Analyses

The next item we assess is whether or not the author's data analyses make sense. We want to know that the author bases the conclusions on adequate data analyses or evaluation of the data. For a very interesting discussion on the term "statistical significance" see Field (2009). In this discussion, Field (2009) mentions an article by Fisher (1956) in which Fisher acknowledged that:

> *No scientific worker has a fixed level of significance at which from year to year, and in all circumstances, he rejects hypotheses; he rather gives his mind to each particular case in the light of the evidence and his ideas.* (Fisher, 1956, as cited by Field, 2009, p. 51)

In other words, "statistically significant" is an arbitrary entity and the magic $p < 0.05$ or $p < 0.01$ are popular trends to report test statistics as being significant at these levels. The most simplistic answer probably is that, during the days before computers, scientists compared their test statistics against published tables of "critical values." It so happened that Fisher, to save space in his far reaching textbook "Statistical methods for research workers" produced only tables for probability values of 0.05, 0.02, and 0.01. So, for no reason other than being readily available, these values encroached themselves on modern statistics as the "gold standard" to report statistically significant results.

The very focus of many peer-review journals on statistical significance might contribute to the file drawer problem or, in other words, reporting bias. This means that research that could inform the field and might be pretty important to move the field ahead, because of the ideas contained will not get published because the results do not show statistical significance. The Cochrane Collaboration writes that publication biases arise when statistically positive results are being "more likely to be published," "more likely to be published rapidly," "more likely to be published in English," "more likely to be published more than once," and "more likely to be cited by others" (Higgins & Green, 2011).

The take home message here is to know that publication bias exists. Here at MindBodyMed Press we focus on the publication of mini-monographs based on sound scientific principles, regardless whether or not statistically significant results are being reported (where applicable).

5. Rationale and Theoretical Development of Hypotheses

Does the author introduce a problem and is it supported by background material? Does the author state the hypothesis or specific question? Is the hypothesis or specific question clearly derivable from theory and/or logically connected to earlier data and arguments? Does the author explain how a particular research design allows the extrapolations needed to scrutinize the hypothesis or the specific question (American Psychological Association, 2010)?

6. Legitimacy of Conclusions

Is the data summarized and adequately analyzed? Is there enough data and in sufficient detail to support the author's conclusion? Did the author attempt to elaborate on all results, even those that were unexpected (American Psychological Association, 2010)?

7. Quality of Discussion

Does the author make, if appropriate, a declarative, and concise assertion of the study results? Does the author elaborate on the meaning of research results and state why these findings are important? Did the author relate findings to similar studies that inspired the author's investigation in the first place? Does the author consider ALL possible explanations rather than only those that fit the author's own biases (Hess, 2004)?

Most importantly, does the author address patients and clinicians by providing at least some context of the findings for the care of patients? Does the author provide some context of the findings for other researchers and to provide suggestions for further study? How about the limitations of the investigation? Simply stated, all studies have limitations, and it is the responsibility of the researcher to point out those limitations and delimitations. Conversely, does the author mention the strengths of the investigation (Hess, 2004)?

8. Conclusion: Contributes New Knowledge to the Field

Here, we look at the "Take-Home Message" of the study. It is essentially an opportunity for the author to elaborate and highlight important points a reader should remember from this mini-monograph (Hess, 2004). The conclusion section also provides an opportunity to provide suggestions for change, if appropriate.

Hess (2004) writes that one should avoid inflating the interpretation of the results, making unwarranted speculations and overly inflating the importance of the findings. It is imperative to stay concentrated on the results, rather than weakening and muddling the real message of the study with tangential hyperbole. Finally, Hess suggests abstaining from using the discussion section to flat-out attack other researchers or "preaching" to the reader and providing conclusions not supported by the data.

Overall Impact and Criterion Scoring

Now that the reader has an idea about **WHAT** we evaluate and analyze when appraising a mini-monograph proposal, it is equally necessary to have an objective rating scheme to evaluate the territory of the eight-fold path network (overall score) as well as the terrain of each distinct path (criterion score)- the **HOW**.

While many methods and schemes exist to evaluate manuscripts, we borrowed and modified a scoring system used by the National Institutes of Health (NIH) to evaluate grant proposals. For the NIH's system, see the document titled "Scoring System and Procedure" (NIH, 2013).

How Does MindBodyMed Press's Scoring System Work?

Overall Impact Score

The overall impact score indicates an appraisal of a project to have a sustained, significant importance on the research fields affected. Reviewers base impact scores on the appraisal of the scored criteria as well as additional criteria. A score can range from one to nine. The score is next multiplied by 10 to decide the final impact score. Thus, the final range of one unique overall impact score for a mini-monograph manuscript is 10 to 90.

Criterion Scoring

The purpose of criterion scoring is to communicate the reviewer's assessment of strengths and weaknesses of individual sections. For criterion scoring, the reviewer gives a score of one to nine along with a written summary critique for each criterion. It must be pointed out that the overall impact score is not the average of the criterion scores.

Reviewer Guidance

The NIH (2013) scoring system and procedure document provides reviewer direction. This material also comprises a table of a score's meaning and description.

Each criterion score, however, should be imposed based on the strength of that particular criterion in the context of the manuscript. It is possible for a reviewer to give only moderate scores to part of the review criteria, yet still give a high overall impact score. This is conceivable because a single review criterion critically vital to the research could be rated high, despite moderate scores being assigned elsewhere, thus giving the whole project a higher impact score (NIH, 2013).

On the other hand, a reviewer might give chiefly high criterion ratings, but rate the overall impact score low, because one criterion critically important to the mini-monograph is not highly rated. The NIH accepts the idea that not all grant applications can or need to be strong in each and every of the evaluation criteria to be still regarded as having excellent overall impact. If this evaluation process is good enough for the NIH (with a 2014 budget of $29.9 billion), it most assuredly merits adoption by an emerging indie publisher such as MindBodyMed Press.

See Table 1 "Guide for Reviewers Assigning Overall Impact Scores and Individual Criterion Scores" on the next page.

While it may be to some extent counterintuitive, the lower the score the better the manuscript. For instance, an overall impact score of 5 is representative of a good, medium-impact mini-monograph.

We must acknowledge that this method is by no means complete or fail safe as a reviewer's personal biases still may find their way into the evaluation process. In spite of that, this process renders a framework that permits individual manuscripts to be appraised based on objective criteria omitting reviewer bias to some degree.

This, in a nutshell, is our evaluation method. Since each manuscript is different, not all forks of the "Eight-Fold Path to a Publishable Mini-Monograph" apply uniformly to all evaluations.

If you are an author thinking about submitting a manuscript, you now have a simple checklist to examine your manuscript as you tailor your document toward publication with MindBodyMed Press.

■ Table 1. Guide for Reviewers Assigning Overall Impact Scores and Individual Criterion Scores		
Overall Impact or Criterion Strength	Score	Descriptor
High	1	Exceptional
	2	Outstanding
	3	Excellent
Medium	4	Very Good
	5	Good
	6	Satisfactory
Low	7	Fair
	8	Marginal
	9	Poor

Note. Adapted from "Scoring System and Procedure" by the National Institutes of Health, 2013, p. 4. Copyright by the National Institutes of Health.

On the other hand, if you are a consumer reading this, you can rest assured that we have taken multiple precautions to report only important, high-quality material, without the hype the latest treatment, miracle cure, and magic pill usually receive and that plaque the field of Complementary and Alternative Medicine.

Thus, MindBodyMed Press pursues its vision of empowering doctors, CAM practitioners, mind-body practitioners, clinicians, and scientists, who are the key holders of knowledge associated with the potential use of mind-body interventions, to provide and share information that is of value to the public.

We believe that making the evaluation process transparent adds value to our mini-monographs and therefore have included the reviewer's comments in the afterword.

Adding transparency to these steps, even though we are not a peer-review journal per se, further positions MindBodyMed Press as a leader in changing the way mind-body scientists, clinicians, and practitioners communicate with the public.

Werner Absenger
Managing Editor and Publisher
MindBodyMed Press
werner@MindBodyMedPress.com

References:

American Psychological Association. (2010). *Publication Manual of the American Psychological Association* (6th ed.). Washington, DC: American Psychological Association.

Field, A. (2009). *Discovering statistics using SPSS: (And sex and drugs and rock "n" roll)* (3rd ed.). London: SAGE.

Gall, M. D., Borg, W. R., & Gall, J. P. (1996). *Education research: An introduction* (6th ed.). White Plains, NY: Longman.

Hess, D. R. (2004). How to write an effective discussion. *Respiratory Care*, 49(10), 1238-41.

Higgins, J. P., & Green, S. (Eds.). (2011). *Cochrane hand-book for systematic reviews of interventions version 5.1.0* [updated March 2011]. The Cochrane Collaboration. Retrieved from www.cochrane-handbook.org

Liberati, A., Altman, D. G., Tetzlaff, J., Mulrow, C., Gotzsche, P. C., Ioannidis, J. P. A., … Moher, D. (2009). The PRISMA statement for reporting systematic reviews and meta-analyses of studies that evaluate healthcare interventions: explanation and elaboration. *BMJ, 339*, b2700–b2700. doi:10.1136/bmj.b2700

Moustakas, C. (1994). *Phenomenological research methods.* Thousand Oaks, CA: Sage.

Scoring system and procedure. (2013, March 25). Retrieved from National Institutes of Health (NIH) website: http://grants.nih.gov/grants/peer/guidelines_general/scoring_system_and_procedure.pdf

Noblit, G. W., & Hare, R. D., (1988). *Meta-ethnography: Synthesizing qualitative studies.* Newbury Park, CA: Sage.

Ogawa, R. T. & Malen, B. (1991). Towards rigor in reviews of multivocal literature: Applying the exploratory case method. *Review of Educational Research, 61,* 265-286.

Literature reviews. (n.d.). Retrieved from University of North Carolina website: https://writingcenter.unc.edu/handouts/literature reviews/

Afterword:

MindBodyMed Press

Manuscript Review

Kathy Blough's The Experience of Being Diagnosed with Cancer

Evaluated by Werner Absenger on March 2, 2014

1. Quality of Design and Methods

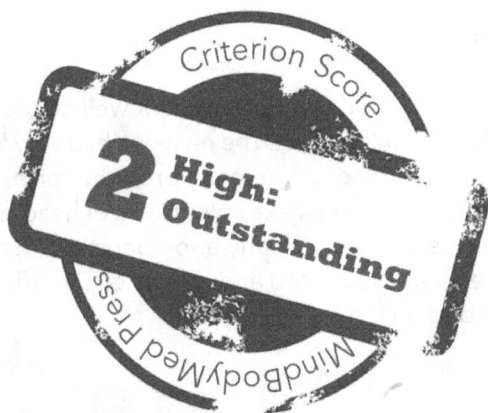

Criterion Score

2 High: Outstanding

MindBodyMed Press

Comments:

Ms. Blough introduces the reader to phenomenological research early and simplifies the process quite well. Ms. Blough guides the reader through the specific steps necessary for the study to be deemed a phenomenological inquiry.

2. Clarity and Readability

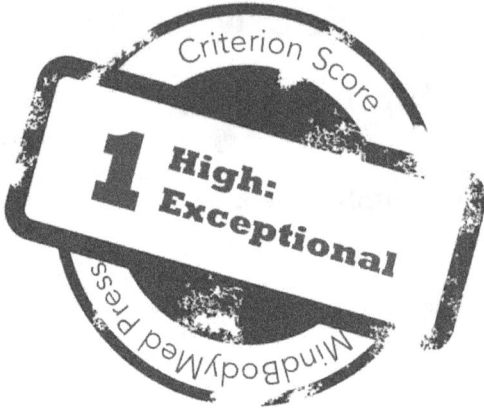

Comments:

The manuscript's length appears well suited to describe Ms. Blough's project. The reviewer had very little difficulty grasping the arguments brought forth by the researcher. Ms. Blough makes plenty use of headings, and she presents concepts clearly and concisely. The manuscript seems well balanced and devoid of superfluous jargon and bias on the author's behalf.

3. Literature Review and Use of References

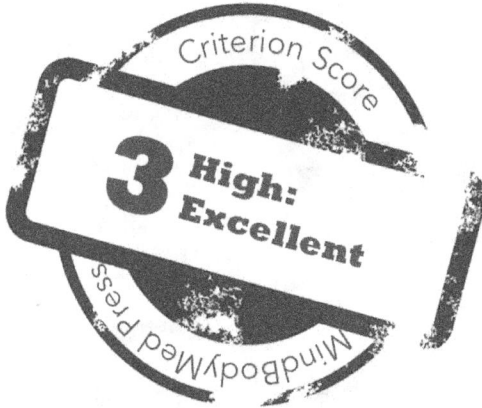

Comments:

While the literature review seems comprehensive and well conducted, the reviewer would have liked supplementary data concerning the databases explored, over what time interval searching the databases took place, as well as precise search terms utilized. This would permit a person interested in researching this subject not only to reproduce this search, but also to spread the search into different databases if appropriate.

Pertaining references: Ms. Blough makes excellent use of references and substantiates the matter with related citations.

4. Adequate Data Analyses

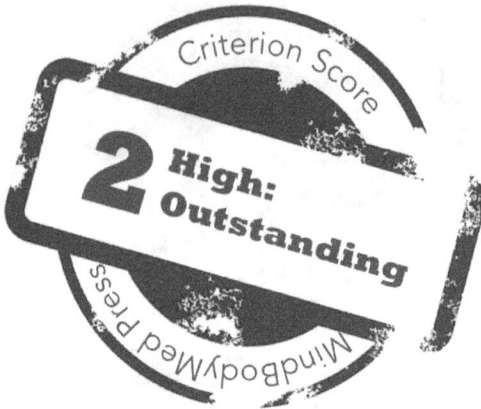

Criterion Score

2 High: Outstanding

MindBodyMed Press

Comments:

Ms. Blough explicitly affirms what sort of data can be extrapolated from phenomenological inquiry. Ms. Blough elucidates her data analysis procedures very well.

5. Rationale and Theoretical Development of Hypotheses

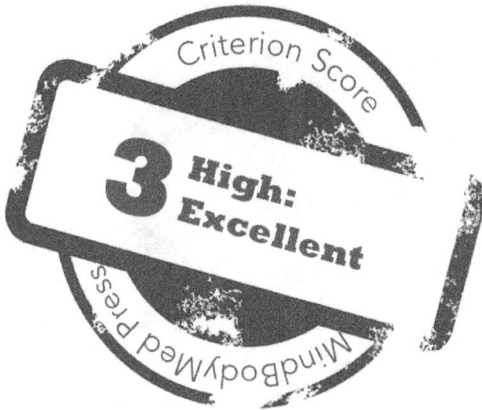

Comments:

Examining the manuscript, the reviewer can readily grasp the rationale of her study. Ms. Blough presents a predicament that demands to be addressed in order to alleviate the pain and suffering of cancer patients. She leaves no doubt as to how the research design permits her to pluck the data to obtain answers to her research question.

6. Legitimacy of Conclusions

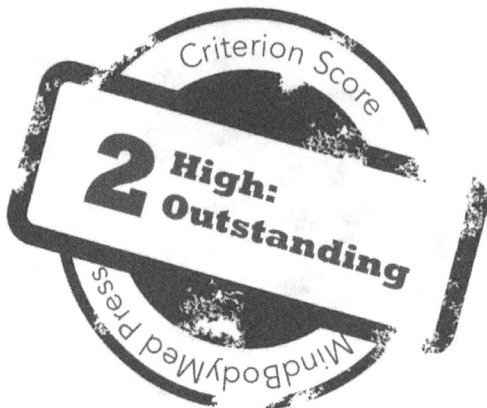

Comments:

The outcomes brought forth by Ms. Blough appear to be well supported by her data analysis. We are presented ample data to surmise that a real problem exists.

7. Quality of Discussion

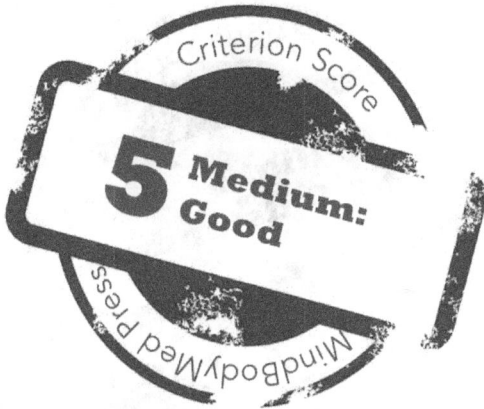

Comments:

While Ms. Blough discusses the need for additional investigation and elaborates on the field of psycho-oncology we are resigned to speculate what type of research might be suitable. One or two distinct research examples would have meant a welcome extension to an otherwise exceptional mini-monograph.

A strength of Ms. Blough's discussion section is that she clearly states the limitations of her study, as well as some strengths of her study. This reviewer would have preferred to have seen a more comprehensive discussion on the distinct strengths of her study. The study design and follow through were meticulous, and as such we discovered a great deal from Ms. Blough's investigation. This fact could have been elaborated on in the discussion section a little further.

8. Contributes to New Knowledge in the Field

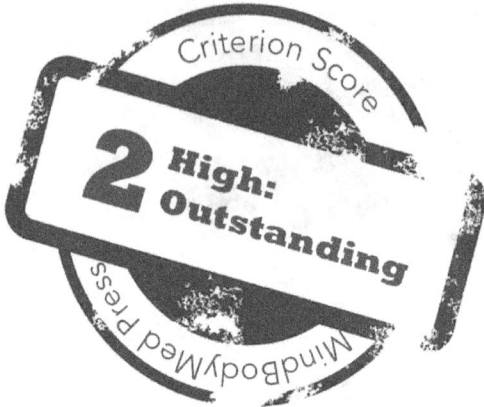

Comments:

Gradually cancer researchers are utilizing psychosocial determinants of the disease and how those factors affect disease outcome. Ms. Blough's research adds a great deal of understanding on the "lived experiences" of cancer patients. Countless cancer patients are not completely certain what to make out of their feelings and emotions. As turns out, addressing the psychosocial factors of cancer might have a concrete bearing on disease outcome.

Overall Mini-Monograph Impact Score

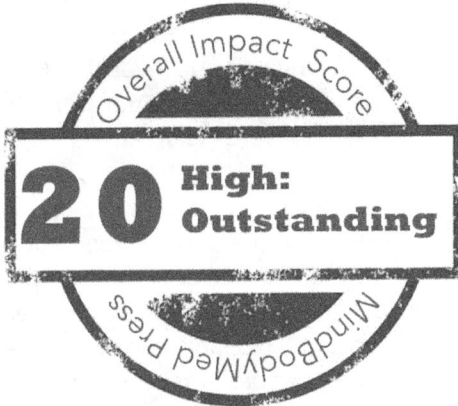

Comments:

Ms. Blough's mini-monograph on the lived experiences of cancer patients is a touching account of three cancer patients as they come to terms with their diagnosis of cancer. Well written and neatly organized, Ms. Blough uses the mini-monograph to guide us skillfully through the turmoil her three co-researchers experience.

Ms. Blough's study was well thought out and executed well adhering to accepted research methods in phenomenological research. The mini-monograph presents with high clarity and is very readable. Ms. Blough bolsters her arguments with a well carried out literature review, and she makes very good use of appropriate references throughout. The data analysis penetrates into "The Experience of Being Diagnosed with Cancer" and supports Ms. Blough's arguments for further research as well as her conclusions.

The rationale and research questions were quite well addressed, leaving no doubt that her model fits the investigation in order to find answers to her question.

Even though this reviewer believes that Ms. Blough's discussion section was a little too brief, contributions of her research to the field were clearly discernable.

Overall, if you are a cancer patient looking for a miracle cure, you will not find it here. However, if you are a cancer patient or loved one/caretaker of a cancer patient who is wondering what you might expect as your cancer journey unfolds, Ms. Blough's research can prove as a valuable starting point to see what psychosocial support and treatments might be available to you.

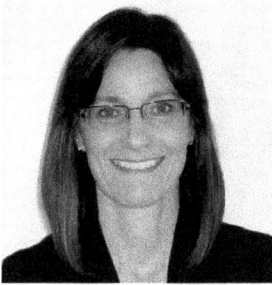

Kathy Blough, PsyS is a Psychotherapist and Certified Holistic Health Counselor. Kathy graduated in 1989 with her master's degree in Clinical and Humanistic Psychology and in 2002 with her specialist's degree in Clinical Psychology and Education. She earned her degrees from the Michigan School of Professional Psychology, in Farmington Hills, Michigan.

In September 2010, Kathy graduated from The Institute of Integrative Nutrition in New York where she became Certified as a Holistic Health Counselor. In 2012, Kathy completed her pilot study, The Experience of Being Diagnosed with Cancer, while pursuing her PhD in Mind-Body Medicine at Saybrook University.

She currently practices psychotherapy and mind-body medicine at her clinic in Ann Arbor, Michigan, Sagepoint Institute for Integrative Health. Reach her at http://www.SPIIH.com/.

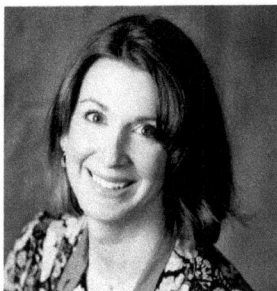

Michele Spilberg Hart, MA, is a freelance editor, non-profit director, and yoga teacher. She graduated from the University of Rochester, Rochester, New York, in 1997 with degrees in Anthropology and Journalism and from Emerson College, Boston, Massachusetts, in 2001 with a Master of Arts degree in Writing & Publishing.

At Emerson she served as head proofreader of the Beacon Street Review. Following graduation Michele edited several medical journals in the Boston area, was on staff as a copy editor at a Boston area paper, and wrote numerous press releases, reviews, articles, and marketing materials for a variety of publications and corporations. She has more than seven years of experience in corporate marketing communications and 10 years working in the non-profit world.

She is also a registered yoga teacher, completing her 200-hour study with Natasha Rizopoulos, as well as Relax and Renew Training with Judith Hanson Lasater, PhD. Michele teaches classes and workshops in the greater Boston area. You can find out more about Michele at www.effortandeaseyoga.com or www.mshmanagement.com.

Thank you for reading!
We invite you to share your thoughts and reactions

Please write a custom review for this title on:

www.MindBodyMedPress.com

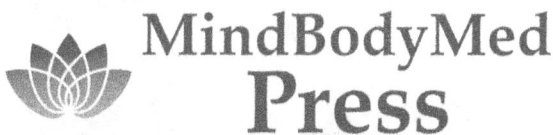

MindBodyMed
Press

Spring Lake | Michigan | United States

Or simply share the title with your friends via:

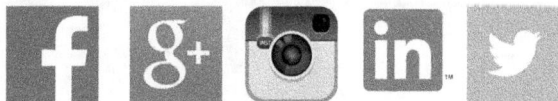